I0469649

On Becoming A Caregiver

On Becoming A Caregiver

Cynthia French
and Bettie Hallett

Copyright © 2011 by Cynthia French and Bettie Hallett

Library of Congress Control Number:		2010918835
ISBN:	Hardcover	978-1-4568-3625-2
	Softcover	978-1-4568-3624-5
	Ebook	978-1-4568-3626-9

All rights reserved. No part of this book may be reproduced or transmitted in any form or by any means, electronic or mechanical, including photocopying, recording, or by any information storage and retrieval system, without permission in writing from the copyright owner.

This book was printed in the United States of America.

To order additional copies of this book, contact:
Xlibris Corporation
1-888-795-4274
www.Xlibris.com
Orders@Xlibris.com
72654

This book is dedicated to Laura Marcinik,
a gracious lady and a very dear friend.

AND

I thank my sister, Carol Becker, and my sons, John
and Tony French, for their continual support and
encouragement as I gathered all my memories for
this book's information.
Cynthia French,
caregiver of many years

I thank Cindy for allowing me to organize, write,
and edit all of her information in this project of
learning and camaraderie.
Bettie Hallett

Contents

The Job of A Caregiver

What is the job of a caregiver?

This is a simple question, and it has a simple answer.

The job of a caregiver is to see that the patient has professional medical attention when needed.

1. The caregiver must know the patient's decisions on his Advanced Health Care Directive, and **protect his rights** by seeing that his wishes are followed.
2. The caregiver is to see that the patient's **physical needs** are taken care of properly by **medical professionals, and only medical professionals**.

Aunt Betty's Advice

Cindy tells that when she took her first summer job, with the lady next door, her Aunt Betty gave her some advice that has served her well over the length of her career.

Aunt Betty told Cindy, "When you go into someone else's home, you do things their way, because you are in their home. Don't try to tell them how you do something. It is their house, and you are a guest in their home. You must respect them and their ways of doing things."

Aunt Betty continued, "Doing things their way makes them more comfortable with you. If you try to push your ways on them, in their own home, they will feel that you are being rude to them and will not like you. The people who live in that home will think you are a 'pushy know-it-all.'

However, if you show respect for their ways, in their home, and ask them how to do things as they would like, they will like you because you are showing them respect and also politely respecting the fact that you are in THEIR HOME," sighed Aunt Betty.

THIS IS VERY IMPORTANT.

AUNT BETTY WAS A VERY WISE WOMAN.

Certification Requirements

The three requirements asked for by all our fifty states are:

1. Red Cross First Aid Certification—renew every two years.
2. Red Cross Adult CPR Certification—renew every two years.
3. High School Diploma

Along with these three established requirements, each state may have more on their requirements for attaining a caregiver certificate. And, you might find that within each state, different counties may also add more items to the established requirements.

To find out exactly what you need, for your local area, contact the local Red Cross. You can call, go to their facility, or go online to find out exactly what requirements you need for certification in your location. The Red Cross is your best source for information about the classes required in your location and where you will find the schools that give these classes.

For your first employment as a caregiver, working for an agency can give a good introduction to the profession. When deciding which agency to use, it is wise to ask a working, experienced caregiver in your area. If you are new to the area and do not know anyone, try going to a hospital and asking the nurses in different areas of the hospital. They usually are full of good information about medical education in the area. They might introduce you to some caregivers that are working in their hospital at that very moment They will also let you know which agency seems to have the most efficient and knowledgeable caregivers.

If you are going to work for an agency, you can contact the agency you are interested in and ask them for their list of requirements. They may send you to the Red Cross for some of the classes, and/or they may offer the classes at the agency.

American Red Cross: 1-800-RED CROSS. *www.redcross.org*

ADVANCED HEALTH CARE DIRECTIVE

An Advanced Health Care Directive states what the patient wants done when he is very ill and cannot voice his decision. So the patient gives the directions in advance of this time. The directions are usually the patient's request not to be resuscitated or to be resuscitated. To protect yourself, make sure the signed form has been legally notarized. This is because *your legal duty is to see that your patient's wishes are respected.*

You must know and understand what your patient has legally directed for his personal health care.

A notary public is a person who has had a clean legal background as checked by the Federal Department of Justice (FBI), has passed the California State Notary Public Certification Examination and has California State Notary Public Certificate, a Notary Stamp and Notary Journal The journal entries keep an exact record of all services rendered by the notary public. The stamp is their personal stamp for use on documents on which they are authorizing the signature. The notary public then affixes his signature on his stamp. And, the two witnesses also sign the document and the notary's journal. The person whose signature is being authorized then signs in the notary public's journal and puts his thumbprint next to his signature. The signed notary public's stamp next to the signature of your patient assures you that your patient's signature is authentic. To protect yourself, you need to know that the signature of you patient is authentic.

If your patient is in a hospital or convalescence home, the facility will have a copy of the AHCD in the patient's file. Ask for a copy for your notebook.

If you are working in a hospital or convalescence home, the staff will take care of seeing that the AHCD instructions are followed. You never make any decisions. Only medical people are legally able to decide what is necessary to do to follow the AHCD.

Keep a copy of the AHCD in the front of your notebook, and make sure you know where it is and what it says.

The doctors and other medical staff members make the final decision. Therefore, your job is to show them your copy of the Advance Health Care Directive—if requested, *but* let them know your patient's wishes about being resuscitated. *Your job is to see that your patient's wishes are respected. And, that is all.*

If you are working in a residence, and you need help, call 911, and have the AHCD in your hand when they arrive so they can read it. Again, you are not a medical person, and under no circumstance are you to make any medical decisions regarding the AHCD.

Keeping your patient's AHCD, knowing what it says and getting help for your patient from medical personnel is you legal responsibility and job

Legal Duties of a Caregiver

CALL FOR HELP

It is extremely important that you, as a caregiver, never take it upon yourself to give medical care that has not been directed or ordered by medical personnel.

When you are working in a hospital or a convalescence home, if you have a problem, help is available immediately. You let the medical staff decide what to do, **ALWAYS. Stay out of their way and when the emergency is over call the person you are to call first.**

When you are working in a residence and there is no one but you with the patient. The only decision you can make is—**who to call.**

If in doubt call 911

Call 911—If you think it might be an emergency.

Have a copy of your patient's AHCD ready for the EMT's.

The EMT's will read the AHCD, and decide if they will take the patient to the hospital.

When the decision has been made by the EMT's, you call the first person on your list and tell them what happened, what the EMT's have decided to do, and ask what the person wants you to do.

If your decision is that this is just a little problem, call the hospice nurse, if that is available to you.

Or call the doctor's office and they will refer you to an emergency number that may be 911.

Your job, as a caregiver, is to make sure your patient receives proper care from medical professionals. That is your legal job.

Professional Insurances

To protect yourself, your family, and your assets, please make sure you are protected by the insurance policies recommended or required for caregivers.

If you need help and advice, consult any agency where you may work and/or an experienced working professional caregiver in your area.

It is recommended, and may be required, that a caregiver have professional liability insurance and workers' compensation insurance. Many employers may require that you have these two insurance policies. Some states, or even different areas within one state, may also require these policies.

You should take this topic seriously, as, without proper insurance coverage, you could find yourself with some serious legal problems.

These topics are fully discussed:

I.   Professional Liability Insurance
II. Workers' Compensation Insurance
III. Income Protection Insurance
IV. How and Where to Purchase Insurance Policies

Professional Liability Insurance

Professional liability insurance is to help protect your rights if you are accused of any negligence that might have caused injury or harm to your patient.

A. If You Are Self-Employed

This insurance is most important, as the patient or his legal conservators have the right to sue you for negligence—if harm or injury to your patient is due to your negligence—or if they think it was your negligence. The patient or his conservator can take you to court to prove their case, and you may need to hire a defense attorney.

If the court finds that you were negligent and caused harm or injury, the court can order you to pay money to the patient for pain and suffering. *Professional liability insurance* protects your interests, hires an attorney and fights for your rights. This type of policy can have many different clauses or parts. Professional liability insurance policies vary tremendously. Take this seriously, and get some good educated local advice about this insurance. Go to agencies and local working caregivers to ask what coverage is recommended and what insurance company or agent they recommend you see. Don't forget the Red Cross.

B. If You Work for an Agency

If you are an employee of an agency, you may find that the agency has professional liability insurance that covers their employees. However, find out about the coverage, so you will know what you can depend on.

Most agencies require their employees to purchase professional liability and workman's compensation policies. They usually let you pay for it every month with money from your earnings. However, find out about the coverage so you will know what you can depend on, if you run into trouble.

You may decide to purchase your own policy *to make sure you have full coverage*.

Again, you may find the best advice from an experienced *caregiver*.

Workers' Compensation Insurance

Workers' compensation insurance is the insurance that covers you when you are injured while on the job and cannot work.

Working for an Agency

When you are working for an agency, they make sure you have this insurance. Each agency may do this in a different way, but you will be aware of the insurance and know that you have a policy in your name.

The agency may carry professional liability insurance for the agency only. This is to protect their assets if one of their employees has a legal liability problem. Check this out carefully, as this could be limited coverage for you. Then you could run into trouble, if a problem arises.

Working for Yourself as an Independent Contractor

If you do not work for an agency, but work as an independent caregiver, you will have to buy your own policy.

When you are hired to be a caregiver for a person who is already admitted to a hospital or convalescence home, you must have your own insurance. Remember, you are not hired by the facility and are not on their staff. Therefore, you are not covered by any of the facility's insurances.

If You Are Going to Work in a Residence

Many people who hire a caregiver think that their home owner's insurance policy will cover a caregiver, if they are hurt in their home. They honestly think this is true.

HOWEVER,—CHECK IT OUT!

Usually this is *not true* for a person *who is hired* to work in or about the house.

1. Home Owner's Policy: This policy usually covers the house and the contents of the home. It *may* also have coverage for a *guest who is hurt* in the home. *But* most likely, it will not have coverage for a person who is hired to work in or about the house. You must check with their insurance agent to find out if you are covered, since you are a hired person in the home.
2. A Renter's Policy: This is a policy that usually only covers the contents of the rented space. Rarely will this have coverage for hired help.
3. The patient or the patient's legal conservator may purchase workers' compensation insurance policy specifically for the patient's caregiver. Check with the insurance agent to make sure you are personally covered by the policy and ask about the coverage. The policy may need your name on it. Find out.

The Benefits That May Be in Your Policy

A. Workers' compensation insurance policies may have many different and varying benefits. You want to know what is in your policy, so you will know what you can depend on, if you are hurt *How are the Costs Covered?*

Workers' compensation insurance policies vary greatly in how they cover medical costs. You must look for this information in the policies:

1. **Does** the policy only give a set amount of money per injury: what is the amount?
2. Does the policy only pay a percentage of the costs?—up to what limit?
3. Does the policy only cover their doctors, chiropractors, dentists, physical therapy, convalescence, etc.
4. Does the insurance company pay the doctor directly?
5. Does the insurance company send you a percentage of the bill, and you are responsible to pay the doctor for the rest of the bill?
6. Look and see if the policy has a limit amount it will pay during one year
7. Does the insurance company only refer you to their doctors?
8. Look at the policy to see how they cover your medical costs.

B. Hospitalization

1. Does the policy pay for an emergency room visit and/or a hospital stay?
2. Again, look at the policy to see if they pay the full bill, only a set amount of the bill, or only a percentage of the bill.
3. Is there is a limit, they will pay for hospital and the doctor's visits? Clarify this information so you aren't surprised with a big bill.

C. Convalescence

1. Look carefully to see if a stay in a convalescence facility is covered.
2. If convalescence is covered, what is the length of stay covered and at what cost to you?

D. Physical Therapy

1. If the policy covers physical therapy, what is the length of coverage, and how is it paid?

E. At-Home Care

1. This is rarely covered, but look and see.
2. And, if your policy has this benefit, look for the limitations and conditions.

F. Lost Wages Benefit

1. Very few policies have this benefit, but you could be a lucky one. *If this is an important item for you*, you may want to see an insurance agent and buy your own income protection insurance policy.

G. Medical Doctors

1. The policy may have provisions to allow you to see your personal doctor, or it may require that you see one of their care providers. Check this out.

2.   The policy *may allow you to use your own doctor, but* your doctor may not accept working with that insurance company. Find out?

Income Protection Insurance

Income protection insurance helps *if you are injured or ill and cannot work.* This type of insurance, like all the others, may have many differences in coverage. When your wages are important, and you cannot work due to illness or injury, this may be a very important policy for you to have

Things to look for in all income protection policies:

1.   How does the illness or injury *qualify* to receive the benefits?
2.   Do the benefits start with the beginning of the illness or injury, or is there a waiting period?
3.   What is the *maximum amount of money* the insurance company will pay *for each* illness or injury?
4.   How are the benefits dispensed: weekly, biweekly, monthly?
5.   Is there a limit as to how many times you may use the policy in a year?
6.   Is there paperwork you need to complete prior to compensation reimbursement?

Discuss this type of insurance with your insurance agent, and decide what policy would be best for you.

How and Where to Purchase Insurance Policies

There are several places where you can purchase insurance policies, and they vary from state to state.

The usual places to purchase your insurance policies:

A. An agent that represents one or several insurance companies
B. The caregivers agency where you may be employed
C. An insurance company that specializes in insurance policies for people in the medical field: doctors, nurses, and caregivers
D. Google might have some good information, too.

List the items you want covered in the policy you will buy. As you shop, check the coverage in each offered policy against your list. Now you can compare the prices for the same coverage.

Hospice in the United States

Josefina Bautista Magno was born on December 28, 1919, in San Fernando, Pampanga, on Luzon. She received a medical degree from the University of Santo Tomas.

Following her husband's death, she came to the United States to work in the hospitals in Washington, D.C. In 1969, she was assigned to work in the United States Office of the Secretary of Health, Education, and Welfare.

In July 1972, she was diagnosed with breast cancer; and during the radiation treatments, which followed a radical mastectomy, she saw, for the first time, the anguish and the suffering that cancer patients and their families go through.

She left the Office of Health, Education, and Welfare and became an oncologist. When Georgetown University Medical Center in Washington, D.C, opened its Division of Medical Oncology, she became one of the first four fellows to train in Georgetown.

It was in the course of her training that she found the need for hospice. Hospice care is the service of offering palliative care. That is patient care when the cure of the patient's disease is no longer possible: caring for patients who are terminally ill.

After attending training courses on hospice care in England and Montreal, Dr. Magno developed the "Georgetown University Pilot Project on Hospice Care". It started with only six beds in a nursing home affiliated with Georgetown.

One of the objectives of the Georgetown project was to define the role of insurance providers in the delivery of hospice care. It was for this reason that the data evolved out of the project became useful to the U.S. Congress. It led to *the Social Security Act* being amended to have hospice care reimbursable by Medicare and Medicaid. Private insurers soon followed.

Dr. Magno was the first executive director of the National Hospice Organization of the United States (NHO). The number of hospice programs in the U.S. grew, within three years, from less than one hundred programs to one thousand two hundred programs that covered all fifty states.

A Patient Covered by Hospice

Hospice is an organization that is part of the Social Security system. When a patient has paid into Social Security, he is entitled to benefits from Social Security and is covered by hospice. Remember, this is for palliative care only. MAKE SURE THE PATIENT HAS AN ADVANCED HEALTH CARE DIRECTIVE.

When a patient is in a hospital, or convalescence home, that facility will have contacted hospice, and a social worker will have been assigned to the patient. The social worker arranges for a hospice nurse to check in on the patient on a regular schedule. The hospice nurse checks to see that the doctor's orders are being followed.

Therefore, when a patient goes home from a hospital or convalescence home, a hospice nurse and the a team of a social worker, a Home Health Aide, a volunteer and a chaplain are already assigned to the patient. The hospice nurse continues to see the patient on a regular basis in his residence, and she also brings some of the medical supplies needed for home care.

A Caregiver's Notebook

The first tool you'll need as a caregiver is your notebook. This will go with you on every job, and is usually the first thing you put into your tote bag. Obtain a three-ring notebook, a package of at least five notebook dividers, a package of five pockets, and one package of lined paper. Yes, like the things you used in high school. This will be one of your most useful tools.

Your notebook must be neat, orderly and up to the minute. It is the first item the doctors and nurses will want to see when they come to visit. Your notebook will tell them: the condition of the patient, hour by hour, the activities (walking—speed, distance, and balance, sitting up alone or with help, and how long), what he ate and the amounts, his pulse, his heart rate, his blood pressure, his medications and dosages, breathing problems, and any other items the doctor has requested. You will also keep all of these items by the time of the day. Ask the doctors if they prefer you use the twelve hour or the twenty-four hour clock.

The first section is for:

In case of emergency.

- You will need the names and phone numbers, in order of calling the patients family

- *This list will be longer when you are caretaking in a residence.*
- *When you are working in a hospital or a convalescence home, this list will most likely be the numbers of the relatives and friends.*
- As you ask for this information, also find out the order in which you should call to tell of problems. This is important
- Family members phone numbers, *the conservator or close family friends*
- All of these numbers must be written in order of who you call first. In other words, *you write them in the order of calling.* Also, it is important you find out who is family, who is a friend, and with *whom you may discuss the patient's health.*

The second section is for :

Medical directives.

- List of medications: time and dosage of each medication
- List of foods appropriate for the patient Daily schedule of activities for your patient
- *You will find an example of a schedule on the next page.*

The third section is for:

Daily records of vital signs and other needed info.

- Make a chart for all of this information. Have several copies of the form you like to use. You have the notebook paper to use to find the schedule you like best. As time goes by, you will find the one that you prefer or make your own. You may even have different preferences for individual patients. Have a page for each day. And keep them up-to-date so if a nurse comes in, she can look at your records and know all of his actions of the day. Take this with you to any doctor's appointments.

The fourth section is for:

Information you must know about the patient.

• Using your notebook paper, write down things you have learned about your patient that will help you. Some examples are: favorite television programs, foods, snacks, sports, favorite games, subjects he enjoys talking about things, subjects he shies away from, his favorite people, hobbies, and books he likes to read.

The fifth section is for pockets to insert necessary documents.

First pocket—**Advanced Health Care Directive**

• You will know what you want in the other pockets as you learn more about your patient. You may fill these pockets with different bits of information for each individual patient.

Examples of column headings for your Vital Signs Page:

Top of one page:		Patient's Name		Day		Date	
Time	Medication	Dosage	How Administered		Alertness	Other Comments	

Personal Items Always With You

When you are a caregiver, you will want some personal items with you, no matter where you are on duty.

Picture the place where your things will be kept. Then pack according to what will fit in the space.

This is a simple list of items that Cindy likes to have with her.

Pack in a soft sided bag, so it can squeeze into spaces.

Personal hygiene items

Change of clothes for three days

Sheet, blanket, pillow, her own pillow case

You may be sleeping in a chair

Booties or slippers

A lounger for sleeping, because in the middle of the night you might have to go to your patient immediately. You must be dressed for work. Or, just sleep in your clothes.

Small camping ice cooler—juices, soda, water, etc.

Food for you. It can very expensive to buy food and drinks at a hospital, and there might not be anything to buy in a convalescence home. In a residence bring your food until you get to know how things work in that residence.

Sweaters, light weight and heavy, so you can layer.

Things you will want to do while the patient is sleeping: knitting, books, electronic games, ear phones for TV, DVD player with ear phones. What you like to do quietly.

Bring some things that you will want to do with your patient to keep him occupied. These items will depend upon the condition of your patient. Ask the patient and his family if they have any ideas.

Relief Time for Caregivers

Hospitals and Convalescence Homes

I. *Work For an Agency:*

When you work for an agency, the agency will arrange the scheduling of the caregivers, and you simply work your shift. Their schedule will have built in relief times. The agency assumes responsibility if a shift is not covered. You simply follow the directives of the agency.

Hospital or Convalescence Facility:

A. *Arrange for relief time*

The family may arrange for a family member or a friend to come and relieve you. Or, the family may feel fine to allow the hospital or convalescence facility staff to be sufficient during your break time. They may want to hire another caregiver and have both of you work to arrange your schedules. Then, make sure this agreement is in writing and signed by all caregivers and the employer This is to protect you and avoid disagreements. This also protects you if something happens during your time off. You want any arrangements in writing and signed by the person or persons who employ you.

B. If Hospice is part of the patient's care, make sure you know when the Hospice person will visit the patient, so you schedule your time to be there. This is important for you. You give a report to the Hospice person, and you may receive some different instructions from the Hospice person. Get all the new instructions from Hospice, or a visiting nurse, in writing for you, the family, employer and the doctor. This is for your protection.

II. Self Employed:

When you are a self-employed caregiver, you must arrange for your own relief time. A good time to do this is when you are interviewing for the position. Make the arrangements for your relief time, and put this schedule in writing with the employer and both of you signing it. Then each of you will have a copy, and this will make times easier for both sides.

Responsibilities In A Hospital

A hospital carries Workers' Compensation Insurance and Liability Insurance for their hired staff. Since you do not work for the hospital, the hospital's Board of Directors will not allow you to work in the facility, as you are not covered by their insurances. (So—Do you have insurance to cover you???) When working for a private patient in the hospital, you will have to buy your personal insurance policies.

When working for a private patient in the hospital you will be very limited as to what you may and may not do.

Obtain all the necessary information you need for your notebook: a copy of the AHCD, the name of the person you will report to and call first, names and phone numbers of family members and close friends and any other information you need to allow you to meet your responsibilities. Take care to be tender and very kind with the patient's family, as they may be very stressed and need your comfort and care, just as your patient does. Be a caregiver to them, too.

Caregivers' Responsibilities To The Patient

Your responsibility, when working in a hospital, is to watch your patient and make sure that help is at his side immediately, if needed. You could go to the nurses' station, on the run if needed, to get help. However, discuss this with the nurses who tend to your patient, and ask them how they would like you to reach them for immediate help. Then follow their instructions.

Follow all of directions given to you by the hospital staff, and tell them how much you appreciate them. Let them know that you have noticed how gentle they are in tending to your patient's needs. When the hospital staff knows you are there only to watch and learn from them, they will be pleasant to your patient, his family and you. Remember, you may not do anything to help your patient physically because of the insurances. Ask the head nurse, on each shift, if you may help feed and give water to you patient. Ask her if she can put that in the chart, so you will have proof of the permission.

Helping Your Patient in a Hospital

Quietly watch closely as the staff turns your patient, and help, if they want your help. As your patient is moved, bathed, changed, etc., you look for any red spots on his back, tail bone, back bone, shoulders, hips, elbows, heels, etc. as these red spots could turn into bed sores. If you see any red spots, carefully, ask the attending staff how are they treating them. Don't use an accusing voice, only a quiet curious voice. You want the red areas treated. Ask if they can be noted in the patient's record, so the doctor will be aware of them. Keep letting the staff know how you appreciate their kindness. However, sometimes the staff will welcome a little of your help and ask you to help them. Use your judgment as to what you will do. Remember, you are not on the hospital's liability insurance or their workers' compensation insurance If allowed, you may help feed your patient and give him water. However, your real job is to observe your patient and keep him occupied. Ask the patient what he would like to do and talk to the family members for some more ideas. Depending on the condition of your patient, try to find a variety of outlets. Write down your ideas in your notebook.

Responsibilities In A Convalescence Home

A Convalescence Home carries Workers' Compensation Insurance and Liability Insurance for their hired staff. Since you do not work for the Convalescence Home, the home's Board of Directors cannot allow you to work in the facility, as you are not covered by their insurances. (SO—Do you have insurance to cover you???) When working for a private patient in a convalescence home, you will have to buy your personal insurance policies.

While working for your private patient, and in the Convalescence Home, you will be very limited as to what you may and may not do.

Obtain all the necessary information you need for your notebook: a copy of the AHCD, the name of the person you will report to and call first, names and phone numbers of family members and close friends and any other information you need to allow you to meet your responsibilities. Take care to be tender and very kind with the patient's family, as they may be very stressed and need your comfort and care, just as your patient does. Be a caregiver to them, too.

Caregivers Responsibilities in a Convalescence Home

Your responsibility, when working in a convalescence home, is to watch your patient and make sure that help is at his side immediately, if needed.

You could go to the nurses' station, on the run if needed, to get help. However, discuss this with the nurses that tend to your patient, and ask them how they would like you to reach them for immediate help. Then, follow their instructions.

Follow all of directions given to you by the home's staff, and tell them how much you appreciate them. Let them know that you have noticed how gentle they are in tending to your patient's needs. When the home's staff knows you are there only to watch and learn from them, they will be pleasant to your patient, his family and you. Remember, you may not do anything to help your patient physically, because of the insurances. Ask the head nurse, on each shift, if you may help feed and give water to your patient. Ask her if she can put that in the chart, so you will have proof of the permission. Sometimes, the staff of a convalescence home will gladly like you help with some things. You be careful! You can help them change a bed or such, but let them hold the patient. If anyone drops or hurts the patient, let it be the person on the staff, not you. But, more often than in a hospital, convalescence home staffs will let you help them and appreciate the help.

Helping Your Patient in a Convalescence Home

Quietly watch closely as the staff turns your patient, and help, if they want your help. As your patient is moved, bathed, changed, etc., you look for any red spots on his back, tail bone, back bone, shoulders, hips, elbows, heels, etc. as these red spots could turn into bed sores. If you see any red spots, carefully, ask the attending staff how are they treating them.

Don't use an accusing voice, only a quiet curious voice. You want the red areas treated. Ask if they can be noted in the patient's record, so the doctor will be aware of them. Keep letting the staff know how you appreciate their kindness. However, sometimes the staff will welcome a little of your help and ask you to help them. Use your judgment as to what you will do. Remember, you are not on the home's liability insurance or their worker's compensation insurance.

Responsibilities in a Residence

We recommend that a caregiver have a least four to five years experience working with an agency before taking a job as the sole caregiver in a residence. As the sole caregiver, everything about the care is up to one person, **you!**

Most people who have home owner's insurance honestly think that you will be covered by their home owner's insurance for injury. **You will not be covered by their home owner's insurance, because you are not a guest, you are hired help.** Therefore, you must make sure you have the proper insurance policies: workers' compensation and liability. If you do not have liability insurance and an injury happens **to your patient,** the patient, his family or his conservator may sue you. You could lose any assets you own.

The caregiver in a residence must be completely proficient with: professional insurances, all of the necessary medicines, the correct dosages of all the medicines, all of the supplies necessary, be able to fully care for the patient's physical and mental conditions, direct furniture placement in the patient's room and have all the information in "the notebook" correct and complete.

If your patient is coming home from a convalescence home or hospital and is palliative, the hospice team assigned will help with many of the supplies. The hospice nurse will be your main contact for medical help with the patient. If you need help with medicines, need to do something that is not in the doctor's directives or have questions, call the hospice nurse (24/7).

However, if there is a problem of a serious nature, call 911. Have the patient's AHCD available when the EMTs arrive. They make all of the decisions. They are the medical people in charge, and you let them do their job. When you know what is going to happen, you call the first person in charge of your patient. You explain what has happened and ask that person what they want you to do. Unless the person asks you to call others, you let that person notify the other people and you follow his/her directions.

If you are alone with the patient and have called hospice for advice or help, and that was enough to solve the problem, call the person who is in charge. Let them know what happened, who you called for advice, describe the directions you followed and assure them that all is fine. This is to always keep the person in charge informed about the patient. Make sure you up-date the incident in the notebook.

Don't let this list of items that Cindy has gathered over many years scare you. The following is a list of the items she keeps in the back of her van. During your practice as a caregiver, you, too, will collect many items, maybe even more then Cindy has.

Patient's Room Arrangement

When being a caregiver in a hospital or convalescence home, the work is easier than working in a residence. This is because of the bedroom furniture arrangement and clutter.

A hospital bed is set with the head of the bed up against a wall. This is allowable, in these facilities, because the bed has wheels and can be moved away from the wall. When you are working in a facility and are not alone, if moving the bed is difficult, you can ask for help. However, when you are the only one in a residence, with no extra help, a bed that has no wheels and is hard to move, moving the bed might be impossible.

There are times when having the head of the patient's bed away from the wall is necessary, as, there are times when the caregiver needs access behind the head of the bed. The caregiver should be behind the head of the patient to allow the use of a pull sheet in pulling the patient gently up in the bed, and there are many unforeseen times when having access to the head of the bed might be beneficial. Since moving the bed in a residence is usually very difficult, we suggest that you arrange the bed away from the wall before the patient gets in it, and leave it there.

You must arrange a clear, unobstructed path from the door to the patient and all the needed supplies.

There must be clear, clean surfaces where the supplies can be kept. These supplies must be in reach while you are attending the patient. Not all of the supplies must be on top of the clean, clear surfaces, only enough to serve you as needed, and the rest may be placed close by, and out of the way. As you use the supplies, simply replace them from the stored ones.

It is suggested that you keep plastic trash bags, of different sizes, by the bed, or even tucked discretely in the end of the bed, so you can grab one or two if needed, for a sudden mess. Cindy recommends that you have at least two or three pairs of disposable gloves in your pockets. You never know exactly when and how quickly you may need to use them.

Cindy also recommends that you buy your disposable gloves a size **larger** then you need. This allows you to put them on very quickly.

Try to have a comfortable chair near the patient's bed to allow normal conversation and comfortable access to each other.

Bedroom Furniture in a Residence

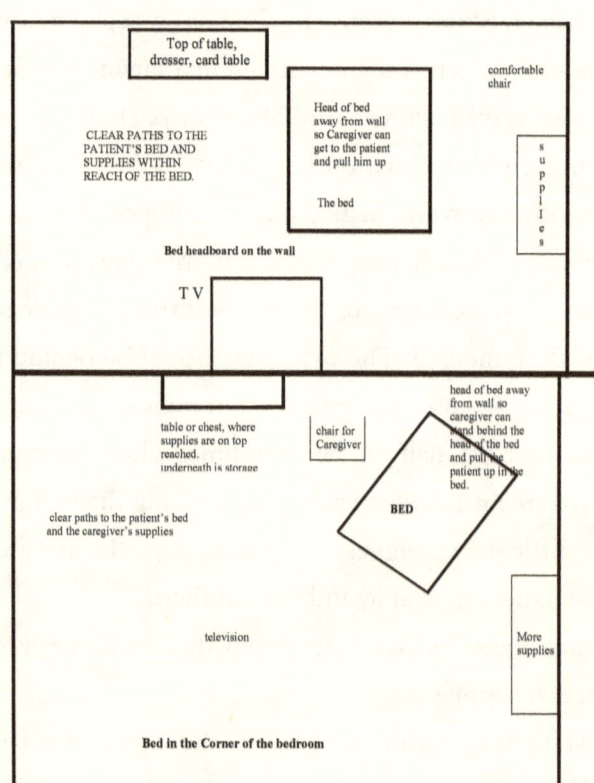

Your Supplies For A Residence

Don't let this list of items that Cindy has gathered over many years scare you. The following is a list of the items she keeps in the back of her van. During your practice as a caregiver, you, too, will collect many items, maybe even more then Cindy has.

1.) Pull sheets—Cindy buys cheap sheets at the second hand stores, and if they are large, she cuts them in half. If they are very thin, she doubles them. As you never want to physically pull, twist or push your patient or hurt your back, a "Pull Sheet" is your miracle tool.

   You can go to the Salvation Army Store, The Goodwill Store or any thrift shop and buy some old sheets. If they are king size, just cut them into three long pieces. After you purchase the old sheet, take them home and wash them in hot water, detergent and Clorox, and rinse twice. Then you can safely use them.

2.) Chucks—Cloth and paper(disposable) chucks are very important to have, especially, if your patient is bed ridden. Again, you can buy very cheap sheets at second hand stores.

3.) Gait Belt—This is a must when you are walking with your patient.
     You can make your own out of rolled up strips of sheeting. Or cut
     old sheets into long strips

4.) Ear thermometer—this is an easy way to take your patient's temperature,
     especially if he is incapacitated.

5.) Blood Pressure cuff—when you purchase one, make sure you calibrate
     it with one in a doctor's office, hospital or at the Red Cross.

6.) Baby medicine dropper—this can be used to give water when the
     patient has a hard time swallowing.

7.) Pill box—this helps organize the medications if they are given more
     than twice a day, or at different times of the day.

8.) Hand sanitizer-have handy if you cannot get to hot water and soap.

9.) Zip lock bags,—to make ice packs if needed for an injury or fever

10.) Baby wipes—for cleaning the patient when needed, Cindy's prefers
     Huggies, as they come out of the box connected evenly

11.) Small paper cups—to put medications in and keep them clean

12.) A baby drinking cup—called a sippy cup—can help give the patient
     liquids when he is sitting up by leaning on an elbow

13.) Baby monitor—to help you when you must leave the room

14.) Flexible straws—helpful with liquids

15.) Pill crusher—small mortar and pistol, to crush a pill if the patient
     cannot swallow the pill. The powder form can be dispensed in liquid
     or apple sauce. The back of a spoon works well sometimes.

16.) A small flashlight—to help check on the patient during the night, and
     see around the room.

17.) Small alarm clock or your cell phone alarm,—to check your patient or
     give medications on schedule

18.) Small circulating fan—when you patient is having trouble breathing,
     using a rotating fan to move the air in the room, may help him breath
     more easily.

19.) Small plastic bottle of water (the short stubby one, 4-6 ounces). With the point of small scissors, poke a hole in the top. Make the hole large enough to put a flex straw through it. Cut the straw to the correct length. Now you can give your patient water when he is down in bed, and this little bottle will fit and stay dry.

20.) Pink Tooth Sponges—these are packaged to be used individually. Put some mouthwash in a small cup and add a little water. Stir with the pink sponges and now use this to swab out the patient's mouth.

21.) **KY Lubrication Gel—use this around the outside and inside of the nose when the patient has an oxygen tube in his nose.** *NOTE; This Gel DOES NOT HAVE OIL IN IT*. **If the lubricating gel has oil in it, and the oxygen leak**s, **the mixture of the oil and oxygen will cause a fire in the patient's nose**.

22.) Loud Bell Where The Patient Can Reach it—This is his way so calling for you. Radio Shack has just come out with a wireless doorbell. You could give the push button part to your patient. As that would take very little energy to push, and keep the bell in your pocket.

23.) Scissors—Scissor are one of your main tools. Your will use a small pair of tending to your patient, another smaller scissors for putting holes in tops of water bottles. You will use the larger scissors for cutting chucks, pull cloths, bandages and other things that come up.

24.) Q-Tips—There are multipurpose to have this item. You will find them handy to have.

25.) Batteries—back up batteries for the baby monitor, your clock, your games, flashlight, radio, portable television, etc.

26.) Small radio with ear phones

27.) Disposable face masks—sometimes the odors can be nauseating, and these help

28.) Safety pins and a Small Sewing Kit—Just sewing a button back on a patient's sleeve or nightgown, makes them feel very special and very happy.

29.) Door Hanger—The little clips that go over the tops of doors and you can hang your clothes on them

30.) Muumuu Nightgowns, or nighttime clothes—so you can come to your patient immediately and still be covered

31.) Disposable trash bags in varying sizes

32.) Disposable gloves, large enough to put on easily. Keep some in your pocket, so you always have some with you.

33.) Alcohol Wipes—These wipes are very helpful in sterilizing tips of things: thermometers, oral or ear, needles, skin areas, etc.

34.) Food Box: Take food for yourself, as you have no idea what the family eats or has on hand. Just keep a plastic box with canned goods, crackers, power bars, juices, a coffee cup and large plastic cups, instant coffee or tea, enough to keep you going for two days, until you can figure out the family food fare.

Part One

Interviewing to Work in a Hospital
or Convalescence Home

The process of interviewing is a two way process. As the person seeking a caregiver is interviewing you, you will also be interviewing the possible employer.

An employer will be looking for a caregiver with the following attributes:

Non-smoker

Soft spoken

Easily understood—does not mumble

Clean hygiene

Short nails that are well manicured

Asks about the patient

Seems to understand some of the patient's problems

Has some questions about things that might have been tried

References from previous employers

What hours you will be able to work

How you would keep the patient involved

This may be some of the information you will want:

What hours do they want you to work

Where will you be working: hospital or convalescence home

How will relief time be arranged and who will relieve you: another
   caregiver, a family member, a friend or the facility staff will be fine
   for your relief time

Who is the single person (the boss) to whom you will answer

What is the salary being paid

As you are talking with the interviewer, think, "Would I like to answer
to this person or work for this person?"

As you enter the building where you might work, check for odors. Some
odors can be very hard to live with. Is there an odor in the patient's room
that you can live with. If not, don't even think about sitting with that odor
for eight to ten hours a day.

Make sure the interviewer takes you to meet the patient. Listen to the way
they speak to each other. Is it a comfortable relationship, or a mean arguing
relationship? Is it a situation in which you could feel comfortable?

Ask where you will sit and have your belongings. If the room does not
smell and looks as though you could spend hours in that chair and be content,
then consider the job. But if you don't think you could stand eight to ten
hours in that chair, in that room, with that patient, then think about it.

Part Two

Interviewing to Be a Caregiver in a Residence

Being a caregiver in a residence is a full time, extremely demanding, job. All of the responsibility for the patient will belong to you. Cindy recommends that you have worked for an agency for at least four or five years before taking on a residential patient. During this training time, you will meet people in your profession. Some of you will become close working associates and friends. You will learn who you can call on in times of need or emergency.

The employer will want you to have a car so you can take the patient places he needs to go.

There will be times when you and one of your friends might be partners as the full time caregivers for one patient. A schedule of the times each of you is on duty is organized. Sharing a patient shows the support and true trust you have in each other as caregivers. Besides friends and trusting colleagues, when working through an agency, your supervisors will learn how families trust you. The members of families will call the agency and request you and tell the supervisor why they want you. These become excellent references for you with your supervisors and the manager of the agency.

When you are ready to be the single caregiver, or have a shared duty caregivers job, in a residence, make sure you have the interview in the residence where you will work.

Besides the interview information given in Part One of Interviewing, you will need to interview for more items, as you will be living in their residence.

Questions you are going to need answered:

Who will you report to?

Who buys the groceries, makes the list, does the cooking?

Where will you park your car, and is it s safe place?

Can I meet the patient and see his room?

Will you be the only one living in the residence with the patient?

Where will you sleep?

Where is your bathroom, or do you share with the patient?

Who does the cleaning other than those of the patient's needs?

If you are going to work there, then you have some things you must discuss with the person in charge.

Show the diagrams of the patient's room arrangement, and discuss this.

You can ask if the family can attend to this, as they know about the furniture in the residence.

Supplies: Does the person in charge know everything that they will need.

Do they have to purchase all the supplies or do they have all the supplies. You have the responsibility of making sure that all the medical supplies you need will be available. But you do not buy them.

Cindy's Antidotes

Dealing With A Patient's Depression

Engage your patient in conversation and listen to him. Conversations about his family, former occupations, hobbies, home, and friends, etc., will help avoid patient depression. Learn things the patient likes to do that can be done while you are with him. Remember to ask your patient, his family and visitors for some ideas. Sometimes you can learn about card games, reading the newspaper, you read to him or he likes to read. Remember to engage him in conversations to show you are interested in him and to let him know that he is important. The patient must feel like a viable person and not just a "thing," laying bed. You, as his caregiver, are a major part of how he feels about himself in this his situation. Do all you can to avoid patient depression by paying attention to him and keeping him busy. Try get him to laugh with you. Laughter is a great help

Dealing with Uncooperative Patients and/or Family Members

When you come across a patient who is giving you problems, I have found that speaking to the person in charge of his care, usually has many good ideas. Most often, the family has been working with this person for a while before you came along to handle him. The family, and also fellow

Caregivers, are good sources for more ideas. Also speak to the patient and ask why he is acting that way. Could be it is the only way he knows how to get attention. Use all the resources you have and have it a good learning experience—are you going to win or the problem patient?

Letters of Recommendation

When you have had a good experience on a job, make sure you ask for a Letter of Recommendation. When you are applying for another job, this is one of the best references you can have.

This is a copy of the last one I received.

October 28, 2010

To Whom It May Concern,

I am writing this letter as a recommendation for Cindy French. I have know her for several years, seeing her devotedly and diligently taking care of many of the patients I have had as a hospice social worker. Her compassion in addition to her skills earned my respect.

Cindy also took care of my mother for several weeks while her regular caregiver of six years was on vacation. My mother had severe problems and depended on total care from her caregiver. Cindy was not only able to master my mother's needs, but also showed compassion and devotion as she tended to her.

In conclusion, I would highly recommend Cindy French for any caregiver role. She is able to quickly learn the needs of her patients and goes far beyond with her devotion and kindness. Any family would be blessed to have her care for someone in their family.

Respectfully, Helen Zimmon

Add your letters of recommendation to your notebook.

www.ingramcontent.com/pod-product-compliance
Lightning Source LLC
Chambersburg PA
CBHW021926170526
45157CB00005B/2209